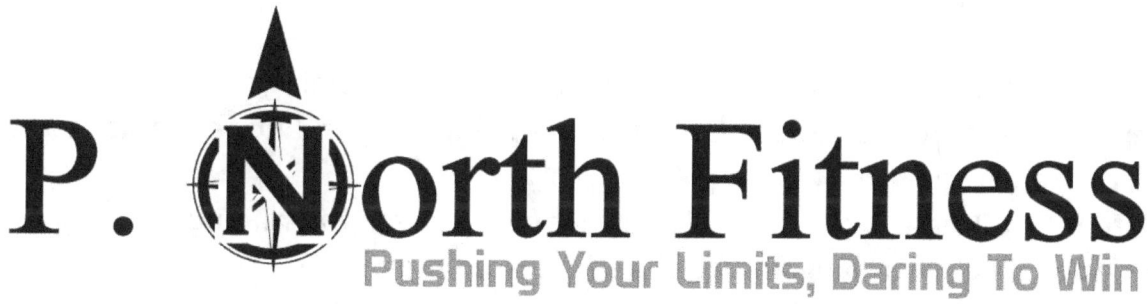

24 Week Fitness Program for Special Forces Selection

This 24 week program will take you from an introductory stage of learning the kind of training methods you will employ to a final testing stage of endurance and strength tests.

This is designed following evaluation of many different Elite and Special Forces tests were evaluated in order to create a plan that can include many methods to prepare you for a wide range of potential regiments.

For this program you will need:

-Military Back Pack
-Access to a gym or Home Weights
-Access to Crossfit
-Access to Swimming Pool
-Weight vests, Military boots and equipment for load training
-Map reading tools

Stage 1- Introductory phase of basic runs and circuit training
Stage 2-1st Progression Phase Circuit training, Running and Rope workouts with basic load carries
Stage 3- 2nd Progression Phase- Circuit Training, Strength Training, Rope workouts, Pack Marching and Assault Circuit training
Stage 4-3rd Progression Phase increases the loads from Stage 3
Stage 5-1st test phase, Endurance test, Combat Swimming Test, Pack March test
Stage 6-Final Endurance Test Week

Stage 1 Week 1
Introduction Stage

Monday
Military Skills Endurance Circuit
Use a trunk, arm and leg format
Circuit 1-Pull Ups

Weighted Sit Up Twists

Body Weight Squats

Circuit 2-Chins

Weighted Sit up Twists

Weighted Step Ups

Circuit 3-Press Ups

Back Extensions

Box Jumps

Perform each exercise to failure 1 minute rest between each circuit, 3 times through the circuit

Tuesday

Rope Workouts with an introduction to climbing techniques

Aim to achieve 3 Rope Climbs

Wednesday

Military Skills Endurance Circuit

Use a trunk, arm and leg format

Circuit 1-Pull Ups

Weighted Sit Up Twists

Body Weight Squats

Circuit 2-Chins

Weighted Sit up Twists

Weighted Step Ups

Circuit 3-Press Ups

Back Extensions

Box Jumps

Perform each exercise to failure reps 1 minute rest between each circuit, 3 times through the circuit

Thursday

20 Minutes swimming in boots, t-shirt and standard combat pants.

Friday

1.5 Mile Run

Saturday

Introduction to training outdoors 1 hour pack march 21lb load

Sunday

1.5 Mile Run

Stage 1 Week 2

Introduction Stage

Monday

Military Skills Endurance Circuit

Use a trunk, arm and leg format

Circuit 1-Pull Ups

Weighted Sit Up Twists

Body Weight Squats

Circuit 2-Chins

Weighted Sit up Twists

Weighted Step Ups

Circuit 3-Press Ups

Back Extensions

Box Jumps

Perform each exercise to failure 1 minute rest between each circuit, 3 times through the circuit

Tuesday

Rope Workouts with an introduction to climbing techniques

Aim to achieve 3 Rope Climbs

Wednesday

Military Skills Circuit

Use a trunk, arm and leg format

Circuit 1-Pull Ups

Weighted Sit Up Twists

Body Weight Squats

Circuit 2-Chins

Weighted Sit up Twists

Weighted Step Ups

Circuit 3-Press Ups

Back Extensions

Box Jumps

Perform each exercise to failure 1 minute rest between each circuit, 3 times through the circuit

Thursday

20 Minutes swimming in boots, t-shirt and standard combat pants.

Friday

1.5 Mile Run

Saturday

Introduction to training outdoors 1 hour pack march 21lb load, use this to learn your pack marching technique and navigation skills

Sunday

MSC Test one rope climb and controlled decent, minimum 3 correct pull ups, level 10 bleep test

Must be passed before progression onto stage 2

Complete wearing combat trousers, belt and service issue boots

Stage 2 Week 1

Progression Stage

Monday

Military Skills Circuit

Use a trunk, arm and leg format

Circuit 1-Pull Ups

Weighted Sit Up Twists

Body Weight Squats

Circuit 2-Chins

Weighted Sit up Twists

Weighted Step Ups

Circuit 3-Press Ups

Back Extensions

Box Jumps

Perform each exercise to failure 1 minute rest between each circuit, 3 times through each circuit

Tuesday

Rope Workouts with an introduction to climbing techniques

Aim to achieve 3 Rope Climbs with a 10lb weight

Wednesday

Military Strength Endurance Training

Warm up with back extensions and running then perform the following with no more than 60 kg weight on the barbell, as many circuits as possible in 30 minutes then onto core work, session should last 45 minutes

Bench Press 10 reps

Military Press 10 reps

Squat 10 reps

Pulls Ups to Failure

Inside Grip Chins to Failure

Dips to Failure

Core Crunches 3x25

Reverse Crunches 3x25

Abs twists 3x25

Thursday

Speed and interval training 1.5 mile with at least 8x100 sprints, preferably up hill

Friday

Military Strength Endurance Training

Warm up with back extensions and running then perform the following with no more than 60 kg weight on the barbell, as many circuits as possible in 30 minutes then onto core work, session should last 45 minutes

Bench Press 10 reps

Military Press 10 reps

Squat 10 reps

Pulls Ups to Failure

Inside Grip Chins to Failure

Dips to Failure

Core Crunches 3x25

Reverse Crunches 3x25

Abs twists 3x25

Saturday

2 Mile Run

Sunday

1 hour pack march 35lb load

Stage 2 Week 2
Progression Stage

Monday
Military Skills Circuit
Use a trunk, arm and leg format
Circuit 1-Pull Ups
> Weighted Sit Up Twists
> Body Weight Squats

Circuit 2-Chins
> Weighted Sit up Twists
> Weighted Step Ups

Circuit 3-Press Ups
> Back Extensions
> Box Jumps

Perform each exercise to failure, 1 minute rest between each circuit, 3 times through each circuit

Tuesday
Rope Workouts with an introduction to climbing techniques
Aim to achieve 3 Rope Climbs with a 15lb weight

Wednesday
Military Strength Endurance Training
Warm up with back extensions and running then perform the following with no more than 60 kg weight on the barbell, as many circuits as possible in 30 minutes then onto core work, session should last 45 minutes
Bench Press 10 reps
Military Press 10 reps
Squat 10 reps
Pulls Ups to Failure
Inside Grip Chins to Failure
Dips to Failure
Core Crunches 3x30
> Reverse Crunches 3x30
> Abs twists 3x30

Thursday
25 Minutes Continuous Swimming

Friday
Military Strength Endurance Training
Warm up with back extensions and running then perform the following with no more than 60 kg weight on the barbell, as many circuits as possible in 30 minutes then onto core work, session should last 45 minutes
Bench Press 10 reps

Military Press 10 reps
Squat 10 reps
Pulls Ups to Failure
Inside Grip Chins to Failure
Dips to Failure
Core Crunches 3x35
    Reverse Crunches 3x35
    Abs twists 3x35
Saturday
2.5 Mile Run
Sunday
1 hour 30 minutes pack march 35lb load

Stage 2 Week 3
Progression Stage

Monday
Military Skills Circuit
Use a trunk, arm and leg format
Circuit 1-Pull Ups
    Weighted Sit Up Twists
    Body Weight Squats
Circuit 2-Chins
    Weighted Sit up Twists
    Weighted Step Ups
Circuit 3-Press Ups
    Back Extensions
    Box Jumps
Perform each exercise to fialure, 1 minute rest between each circuit, 3 times through each circuit
Tuesday
Rope Workouts with an introduction to climbing techniques
Aim to achieve 3 Rope Climbs with a 25lb weight
Wednesday
Military Strength Endurance Training
Warm up with back extensions and running then perform the following with no more than 60 kg weight on the barbell, as many circuits as possible in 30 minutes then onto core work, session should last 45 minutes
Bench Press 10 reps
Military Press 10 reps
Squat 10 reps
Pulls Ups to Failure
Inside Grip Chins to Failure
Dips to Failure
Core Crunches 3x45
    Reverse Crunches 3x45

Abs twists 3x45
Thursday
Speed and interval training 1.5 mile with at least 10x100m sprints, preferably up hill
Friday
Military Strength Endurance Training
Warm up with back extensions and running then perform the following with no more than 60 kg weight on the barbell, as many circuits as possible in 30 minutes then onto core work, session should last 45 minutes
Bench Press 10 reps
Military Press 10 reps
Squat 10 reps
Pulls Ups to Failure
Inside Grip Chins to Failure
Dips to Failure
Core Crunches 3x45
    Reverse Crunches 3x45
    Abs twists 3x45
Saturday
3 Mile Run
Sunday
1 hour 30 minutes pack march 45lb load

Stage 2 Week 4
Progression Stage

Monday
Military Skills Circuit
Use a trunk, arm and leg format
Circuit 1-Pull Ups
    Weighted Sit Up Twists
    Body Weight Squats
Circuit 2-Chins
    Weighted Sit up Twists
    Weighted Step Ups
Circuit 3-Press Ups
    Back Extensions
    Box Jumps
Perform each exercise to failure, 1 minute rest between each circuit, 3 times through each circuit
Tuesday
Rope Workouts with an introduction to climbing techniques
Aim to achieve 3 Rope Climbs with a 35lb weight
Wednesday
Military Strength Endurance Training

Warm up with back extensions and running then perform the following with no more than 60 kg weight on the barbell, as many circuits as possible in 30 minutes then onto core work, session should last 45 minutes

Bench Press 10 reps

Military Press 10 reps

Squat 10 reps

Pulls Ups to Failure

Inside Grip Chins to Failure

Dips to Failure

Core Crunches 3x50

    Reverse Crunches 3x50

    Abs twists 3x50

Thursday

30 Minutes Continuous Swimming

Friday

Military Strength Endurance Training

Warm up with back extensions and running then perform the following with no more than 60 kg weight on the barbell, as many circuits as possible in 30 minutes then onto core work, session should last 45 minutes

Bench Press 10 reps

Military Press 10 reps

Squat 10 reps

Pulls Ups to Failure

Inside Grip Chins to Failure

Dips to Failure

Core Crunches 3x50

    Reverse Crunches 3x50

    Abs twists 3x50

Saturday

3.5 Mile Run

Sunday

1 hour 30 minutes pack march 45lb load

Stage 2 Week 5

Progression Stage

Monday

Military Skills Circuit

Use a trunk, arm and leg format

Circuit 1-Pull Ups

    Weighted Sit Up Twists

    Body Weight Squats

Circuit 2-Chins

    Weighted Sit up Twists

    Weighted Step Ups

Circuit 3-Press Ups

Back Extensions

Box Jumps

Perform each exercise to failure, 1 minute rest between each circuit, 3 times through each circuit

Tuesday

Rope Workouts with an introduction to climbing techniques

Aim to achieve 3 Rope Climbs with a 45lb weight

Wednesday

Military Strength Endurance Training

Warm up with back extensions and running then perform the following with no more than 60 kg weight on the barbell, as many circuits as possible in 30 minutes then onto core work, session should last 45 minutes

Bench Press 10 reps

Military Press 10 reps

Squat 10 reps

Pulls Ups to Failure

Inside Grip Chins to Failure

Dips to Failure

Core Crunches 3x55

    Reverse Crunches 3x55

    Abs twists 3x55

Thursday

1.5 Mile Run 10x100m sprints up hills if possible

Friday

Military Strength Endurance Training

Warm up with back extensions and running then perform the following with no more than 60 kg weight on the barbell, as many circuits as possible in 30 minutes then onto core work, session should last 45 minutes

Bench Press 10 reps

Military Press 10 reps

Squat 10 reps

Pulls Ups to Failure

Inside Grip Chins to Failure

Dips to Failure

Core Crunches 3x50

    Reverse Crunches 3x50

    Abs twists 3x50

Saturday

4 Mile Run

Sunday

1 hour 30 minutes pack march 45lb load

Stage 2 Week 6

Progression Stage

Monday

Military Skills Circuit

Use a trunk, arm and leg format

Circuit 1-Pull Ups

>Weighted Sit Up Twists

>Body Weight Squats

Circuit 2-Chins

>Weighted Sit up Twists

>Weighted Step Ups

Circuit 3-Press Ups

>Back Extensions

>Box Jumps

Perform each exercise to failure, 1 minute rest between each circuit, 3 times through each circuit

Tuesday

Rope Workouts with an introduction to climbing techniques

Aim to achieve 3 Rope Climbs with a 50lb weight

Wednesday

Military Strength Endurance Training

Warm up with back extensions and running then perform the following with no more than 60 kg weight on the barbell, as many circuits as possible in 30 minutes then onto core work, session should last 45 minutes

Bench Press 10 reps

Military Press 10 reps

Squat 10 reps

Pulls Ups to Failure

Inside Grip Chins to Failure

Dips to Failure

Core Crunches 3x55

>Reverse Crunches 3x55

>Abs twists 3x55

Thursday

30 Minutes Continuous Swimming

Friday

Military Strength Endurance Training

Warm up with back extensions and running then perform the following with no more than 60 kg weight on the barbell, as many circuits as possible in 30 minutes then onto core work, session should last 45 minutes

Bench Press 10 reps

Military Press 10 reps

Squat 10 reps

Pulls Ups to Failure

Inside Grip Chins to Failure

Dips to Failure

Core Crunches 3x55

>Reverse Crunches 3x55

>Abs twists 3x55

Saturday

4.5 Mile Run
2 hour pack march 45lb load

Stage 2 Week 7
Progression Stage

Monday
Military Skills Circuit
Use a trunk, arm and leg format
Circuit 1-Pull Ups
       Weighted Sit Up Twists
       Body Weight Squats
Circuit 2-Chins
       Weighted Sit up Twists
       Weighted Step Ups
Circuit 3-Press Ups
       Back Extensions
       Box Jumps
Perform each exercise to failure, 1 minute rest between each circuit, 3 times through each circuit

Tuesday
Rope Workouts with an introduction to climbing techniques
Aim to achieve 3 Rope Climbs with a 55lb weight

Wednesday
Military Strength Endurance Training
Warm up with back extensions and running then perform the following with no more than 60 kg weight on the barbell, as many circuits as possible in 30 minutes then onto core work, session should last 45 minutes
Bench Press 10 reps
Military Press 10 reps
Squat 10 reps
Pulls Ups to Failure
Inside Grip Chins to Failure
Dips to Failure
Core Crunches 3x60
    Reverse Crunches 3x60
    Abs twists 3x60

Thursday
2 mile run with 10x100m sprint up hills if possible

Friday
Military Strength Endurance Training
Warm up with back extensions and running then perform the following with no more than 60 kg weight on the barbell, as many circuits as possible in 30 minutes then onto core work, session should last 45 minutes
Bench Press 10 reps

Military Press 10 reps
Squat 10 reps
Pulls Ups to Failure
Inside Grip Chins to Failure
Dips to Failure
Core Crunches 3x60
    Reverse Crunches 3x60
    Abs twists 3x60

Saturday
5.5 Mile Run
Sunday
2 hour pack march 55lb load

Stage 2 Week 8
Progression Stage

Monday
Military Skills Circuit
Use a trunk, arm and leg format
Circuit 1-Pull Ups
        Weighted Sit Up Twists
        Body Weight Squats
Circuit 2-Chins
        Weighted Sit up Twists
        Weighted Step Ups
Circuit 3-Press Ups
        Back Extensions
        Box Jumps
Perform each exercise to failure, 1 minute rest between each circuit, 3 times through each circuit

Tuesday
Rope Workouts with an introduction to climbing techniques
Aim to achieve 3 Rope Climbs with a 61lb weight
Wednesday
Military Strength Endurance Training
Warm up with back extensions and running then perform the following with no more than 60 kg weight on the barbell, as many circuits as possible in 30 minutes then onto core work, session should last 45 minutes
Bench Press 10 reps
Military Press 10 reps
Squat 10 reps
Pulls Ups to Failure
Inside Grip Chins to Failure
Dips to Failure

Core Crunches 3x65
  Reverse Crunches 3x65
  Abs twists 3x65

Thursday

35 Minutes Continuous Swimming

Friday

Military Strength Endurance Training

Warm up with back extensions and running then perform the following with no more than 60 kg weight on the barbell, as many circuits as possible in 30 minutes then onto core work, session should last 45 minutes

Bench Press 10 reps

Military Press 10 reps

Squat 10 reps

Pulls Ups to Failure

Inside Grip Chins to Failure

Dips to Failure

Core Crunches 3x65
  Reverse Crunches 3x65
  Abs twists 3x65

Saturday

6 Mile Run

Sunday

Stage 2 MSC Test

3 Rope climbs 30lb load and learn to use a makefast technique

5 Full Form Pull Ups

Level 11 on bleep test

Stage 3 Week 9

2nd Progression Stage

Monday

Military Assault Circuit

Weighted Step Ups 3x12

Weighted Lunges 3x12

 Box jumps between two boxes 3x12

Swiss Ball Pike 3x12

Burpee's 3x failure

Bench Press 4x6

Pull Ups x failure

Sprints 45 seconds sprinting with 1 minute rest repeat 8-10 times, rest 1 minute 30 seconds between circuits

Tuesday

Military Strength Endurance Training

Warm up with back extensions and running then perform the following with no more than 60 kg weight on the barbell, as many circuits as possible in 30 minutes then onto core work, session should last 45 minutes

Bench Press 10 reps

Military Press 10 reps

Squat 10 reps

Pulls Ups to Failure

Inside Grip Chins to Failure

Dips to Failure

Core Crunches 4x30

    Reverse Crunches 4x30

    Abs twists 4x30

Wednesday

Endurance pack march 2 hours 30 minutes 55lb load

Thursday

40 Minutes Continuous Swimming

Rope Workouts with an introduction to climbing techniques

Aim to achieve 3 Rope Climbs with a 70lb weight

Friday

Strength Workouts for load carrying and Core strength

1 Mile Run 8 Minute Pace

Dead lift 5 reps

Weighted Glute Ham Raise 5 reps

Weighted Lunges 10 reps

Turkish Get Ups 5 Minutes continuously

Perform the circuit 3-5 times, try and increase weight each week

Saturday

4 mile speed march 40 minutes with 21lb load record your best time

Sunday

6.5 Mile run

Stage 3 Week 10

2nd Progression Stage

Monday

Military Assault Circuit

Weighted Step Ups 3x12

Weighted Lunges 3x12

Box jumps between two boxes 3x12

Swiss Ball Pike 3x12

Burpee's 3x failure

Bench Press 4x6

Pull Ups x failure

Sprints 45 seconds sprinting with 1 minute rest repeat 8-10 times, rest 1 minute 30 seconds between circuits

Tuesday

Military Strength Endurance Training

Warm up with back extensions and running then perform the following with no more than 60 kg weight on the barbell, as many circuits as possible in 30 minutes then onto core work, session should last 45 minutes

Bench Press 10 reps

Military Press 10 reps

Squat 10 reps

Pulls Ups to Failure

Inside Grip Chins to Failure

Dips to Failure

Core Crunches 4x35

    Reverse Crunches 4x35

    Abs twists 4x35

Wednesday

Endurance pack march 2 hours 30 minutes 55lb load

Thursday

45 Minutes Continuous Swimming

Rope Workouts with an introduction to climbing techniques

Aim to achieve 3 Rope Climbs with a 80lb weight

Friday

Strength Workouts for load carrying and Core strength

1 Mile Run 8 Minute Pace

Dead lift 5 reps

Weighted Glute Ham Raise 5 reps

Weighted Lunges 10 reps

Turkish Get Ups 5 Minutes continuously

Perform the circuit 3-5 times, try and increase weight each week

Saturday

4 mile speed march 40 minutes with 21lb load record your best time

Sunday

7 Mile run

Stage 3 Week 11

2nd Progression Stage

Monday

Military Assault Circuit

Weighted Step Ups 3x12

Weighted Lunges 3x12

 Box jumps between two boxes 3x12

Swiss Ball Pike 3x12

Burpee's 3x failure

Bench Press 4x6

Pull Ups x failure

Sprints 45 seconds sprinting with 1 minute rest repeat 8-10 times, rest 1 minute 30 seconds between circuits

Tuesday

Military Strength Endurance Training

Warm up with back extensions and running then perform the following with no more than 60 kg weight on the barbell, as many circuits as possible in 30 minutes then onto core work, session should last 45 minutes

Bench Press 10 reps

Military Press 10 reps

Squat 10 reps

Pulls Ups to Failure

Inside Grip Chins to Failure

Dips to Failure

Core Crunches 4x35

    Reverse Crunches 4x35

    Abs twists 4x35

Wednesday

Endurance pack march 2 hours 30 minutes 61lb load

Thursday

50 Minutes Continuous Swimming

Rope Workouts with an introduction to climbing techniques

Aim to achieve 3 Rope Climbs with a 90lb weight

Friday

Strength Workouts for load carrying and Core strength

1 Mile Run 8 Minute Pace

Dead lift 5 reps

Weighted Glute Ham Raise 5 reps

Weighted Lunges 10 reps

Turkish Get Ups 5 Minutes continuously

Perform the circuit 3-5 times, try and increase weight each week

Saturday

4 mile speed march 40 minutes with 21lb load record your best time

Sunday

7.5 Mile run

Stage 3 Week 12

2nd Progression Stage

Monday

Military Assault Circuit

Weighted Step Ups 3x12

Weighted Lunges 3x12

Box jumps between two boxes 3x12

Swiss Ball Pike 3x12

Burpee's 3x failure

Bench Press 4x6

Pull Ups x failure

Sprints 45 seconds sprinting with 1 minute rest repeat 8-10 times, rest 1 minute 30 seconds between circuits

Tuesday
Military Strength Endurance Training
Warm up with back extensions and running then perform the following with no more than 60 kg weight on the barbell, as many circuits as possible in 30 minutes then onto core work, session should last 45 minutes
Bench Press 10 reps
Military Press 10 reps
Squat 10 reps
Pulls Ups to Failure
Inside Grip Chins to Failure
Dips to Failure
Core Crunches 4x40
    Reverse Crunches 4x40
    Abs twists 4x40

Wednesday
Endurance pack march 2 hours 30 minutes 61lb load

Thursday
55 Minutes Continuous Swimming
Rope Workouts with an introduction to climbing techniques
Aim to achieve 3 Rope Climbs with a 110lb weight

Friday
Strength Workouts for load carrying and Core strength
1 Mile Run 8 Minute Pace
Dead lift 5 reps
Weighted Glute Ham Raise 5 reps
Weighted Lunges 10 reps
Turkish Get Ups 5 Minutes continuously
Perform the circuit 3-5 times, try and increase weight each week

Saturday
4 mile speed march 40 minutes with 21lb load record your best time

Sunday
8 Mile run best effort record your time

Stage 3 Week 13
2nd Progression Stage

Monday
Military Assault Circuit
Weighted Step Ups 3x12
Weighted Lunges 3x12
 Box jumps between two boxes 3x12
Swiss Ball Pike 3x12
Burpee's 3x failure
Bench Press 4x6

Pull Ups x failure

Sprints 45 seconds sprinting with 1 minute rest repeat 8-10 times, rest 1 minute 30 seconds between circuits

Tuesday

Military Strength Endurance Training

Warm up with back extensions and running then perform the following with no more than 60 kg weight on the barbell, as many circuits as possible in 30 minutes then onto core work, session should last 45 minutes

Bench Press 10 reps

Military Press 10 reps

Squat 10 reps

Pulls Ups to Failure

Inside Grip Chins to Failure

Dips to Failure

Core Crunches 4x45

    Reverse Crunches 4x45

    Abs twists 4x45

Wednesday

Endurance pack march 2 hours 30 minutes 61lb load

Thursday

1 Hour Continuous Swimming

Rope Workouts with an introduction to climbing techniques

Aim to achieve 3 Rope Climbs with a 115lb weight

Friday

Strength Workouts for load carrying and Core strength

1 Mile Run 8 Minute Pace

Dead lift 5 reps

Weighted Glute Ham Raise 5 reps

Weighted Lunges 10 reps

Turkish Get Ups 5 Minutes continuously

Perform the circuit 3-5 times, try and increase weight each week

Saturday

4 mile speed march 40 minutes with 21lb load record your best time

Sunday

8 Mile run best effort

Stage 3 Week 14

2nd Progression Stage

Monday

Military Assault Circuit

Weighted Step Ups 3x12

Weighted Lunges 3x12

Box jumps between two boxes 3x12

Swiss Ball Pike 3x12

Burpee's 3x failure

Bench Press 4x6

Pull Ups x failure

Sprints 45 seconds sprinting with 1 minute rest repeat 8-10 times, rest 1 minute 30 seconds between circuits

Tuesday

Military Strength Endurance Training

Warm up with back extensions and running then perform the following with no more than 60 kg weight on the barbell, as many circuits as possible in 30 minutes then onto core work, session should last 45 minutes

Bench Press 10 reps

Military Press 10 reps

Squat 10 reps

Pulls Ups to Failure

Inside Grip Chins to Failure

Dips to Failure

Core Crunches 4x50

    Reverse Crunches 4x50

    Abs twists 4x50

Wednesday

Endurance pack march 2 hours 30 minutes 61lb load

Thursday

1 Hour Continuous Swimming

Rope Workouts with an introduction to climbing techniques

Aim to achieve 3 Rope Climbs with a 125lb weight

Friday

Strength Workouts for load carrying and Core strength

1 Mile Run 8 Minute Pace

Dead lift 5 reps

Weighted Glute Ham Raise 5 reps

Weighted Lunges 10 reps

Turkish Get Ups 5 Minutes continuously

Perform the circuit 3-5 times, try and increase weight each week

Saturday

4 mile speed march 40 minutes with 21lb load record your best time

Sunday

MSC Test

10 strict Pull Ups Minimum

1 Rope climbs 151lb load

12 on the bleep test

Stage 4 Week 15

3rd Progression Stage

Monday

Military Assault Circuit

Weighted Step Ups 3x12

Weighted Lunges 3x12

Box jumps between two boxes 3x12

Swiss Ball Pike 3x12

Burpee's 3x failure

Bench Press 4x6

Pull Ups x failure

Sprints 45 seconds sprinting with 1 minute rest repeat 8-10 times, rest 1 minute 30 seconds between circuits **add a weight vest to you workouts at 10lb weight**

Tuesday

Military Strength Endurance Training

Warm up with back extensions and running then perform the following with no more than 60 kg weight on the barbell, as many circuits as possible in 30 minutes then onto core work, session should last 45 minutes

Bench Press 10 reps

Military Press 10 reps

Squat 10 reps

Pulls Ups to Failure

Inside Grip Chins to Failure

Dips to Failure

Core Crunches 4x55

    Reverse Crunches 4x55

    Abs twists 4x55

Wednesday

Endurance pack march 2 hours 30 minutes 61lb load

Thursday

1 Hour 10 minutes Continuous Swimming

Friday

Strength Workouts for load carrying and Core strength

1 Mile Run 8 Minute Pace

Dead lift 5 reps

Weighted Glute Ham Raise 5 reps

Weighted Lunges 10 reps

Turkish Get Ups 5 Minutes continuously

Perform the circuit 3-5 times, try and increase weight each week increase the load each time

Saturday

6 mile speed march 40 minutes with 21lb load record your best time

Sunday

1 hour speed marching in 31lb load

Stage 4 Week 16

3rd Progression Stage

Monday

Military Assault Circuit

Weighted Step Ups 3x12

Weighted Lunges 3x12

Box jumps between two boxes 3x12

Swiss Ball Pike 3x12

Burpee's 3x failure

Bench Press 4x6

Pull Ups x failure

Sprints 45 seconds sprinting with 1 minute rest repeat 8-10 times, rest 1 minute 30 seconds between circuits **add a weight vest to you workouts at 15lb weight**

Tuesday

Military Strength Endurance Training

Warm up with back extensions and running then perform the following with no more than 60 kg weight on the barbell, as many circuits as possible in 30 minutes then onto core work, session should last 45 minutes

Bench Press 10 reps

Military Press 10 reps

Squat 10 reps

Pulls Ups to Failure

Inside Grip Chins to Failure

Dips to Failure

Core Crunches 4x60

      Reverse Crunches 4x60

      Abs twists 4x60

Wednesday

Endurance pack march 3 hour s 61lb load

Thursday

1 Hour 15 minutes Continuous Swimming

Friday

Strength Workouts for load carrying and Core strength

1 Mile Run 8 Minute Pace

Dead lift 5 reps

Weighted Glute Ham Raise 5 reps

Weighted Lunges 10 reps

Turkish Get Ups 5 Minutes continuously

Perform the circuit 3-5 times, try and increase weight each week increase the load each time

Saturday

6 mile speed march 40 minutes with 21lb load record your best time

Sunday

1 hour speed marching in 31lb load

Stage 4 Week 17

3rd Progression Stage

Monday

Military Assault Circuit

Weighted Step Ups 3x12

Weighted Lunges 3x12

 Box jumps between two boxes 3x12

Swiss Ball Pike 3x12

Burpee's 3x failure

Bench Press 4x6

Pull Ups x failure

Sprints 45 seconds sprinting with 1 minute rest repeat 8-10 times, rest 1 minute 30 seconds between circuits **add a weight vest to you workouts at 15lb weight**

Tuesday

Military Strength Endurance Training

Warm up with back extensions and running then perform the following with no more than 60 kg weight on the barbell, as many circuits as possible in 30 minutes then onto core work, session should last 45 minutes

Bench Press 10 reps

Military Press 10 reps

Squat 10 reps

Pulls Ups to Failure

Inside Grip Chins to Failure

Dips to Failure

Core Crunches 4x65

     Reverse Crunches 4x65

     Abs twists 4x65

Wednesday

Endurance pack march 3 hour s 61lb load

Thursday

1 Hour 20 minutes Continuous Swimming

Friday

Strength Workouts for load carrying and Core strength

1 Mile Run 8 Minute Pace

Dead lift 5 reps

Weighted Glute Ham Raise 5 reps

Weighted Lunges 10 reps

Turkish Get Ups 5 Minutes continuously

Perform the circuit 3-5 times, try and increase weight each week increase the load each time

Saturday

6 mile speed march 40 minutes with 21lb load record your best time

Sunday

1 hour speed marching in 31lb load

Stage 4 Week 18

3rd Progression Stage

Monday

Military Assault Circuit

Weighted Step Ups 3x12

Weighted Lunges 3x12

Box jumps between two boxes 3x12

Swiss Ball Pike 3x12

Burpee's 3x failure

Bench Press 4x6

Pull Ups x failure

Sprints 45 seconds sprinting with 1 minute rest repeat 8-10 times, rest 1 minute 30 seconds between circuits **add a weight vest to you workouts at 21lb weight**

Tuesday

Military Strength Endurance Training

Warm up with back extensions and running then perform the following with no more than 60 kg weight on the barbell, as many circuits as possible in 30 minutes then onto core work, session should last 45 minutes

Bench Press 10 reps

Military Press 10 reps

Squat 10 reps

Pulls Ups to Failure

Inside Grip Chins to Failure

Dips to Failure

Core Crunches 4x70

     Reverse Crunches 4x70

     Abs twists 4x70

Wednesday

Endurance pack march 3 hour 30 Minutes pack march 61lb load

Thursday

1 Hour 30 minutes Continuous Swimming

Friday

Strength Workouts for load carrying and Core strength

1 Mile Run 8 Minute Pace

Dead lift 5 reps

Weighted Glute Ham Raise 5 reps

Weighted Lunges 10 reps

Turkish Get Ups 5 Minutes continuously

Perform the circuit 3-5 times, try and increase weight each week increase the load each time

Saturday

6 mile speed march 40 minutes with 21lb load record your best time

Sunday

1 hour speed marching in 31lb load

Stage 4 Week 19

3rd Progression Stage

Monday

Military Assault Circuit

Weighted Step Ups 3x12

Weighted Lunges 3x12

Box jumps between two boxes 3x12

Swiss Ball Pike 3x12

Burpee's 3x failure

Bench Press 4x6

Pull Ups x failure

Sprints 45 seconds sprinting with 1 minute rest repeat 8-10 times, rest 1 minute 30 seconds between circuits **add a weight vest to you workouts at 30lb weight**

Tuesday

Military Strength Endurance Training

Warm up with back extensions and running then perform the following with no more than 60 kg weight on the barbell, as many circuits as possible in 30 minutes then onto core work, session should last 45 minutes

Bench Press 10 reps

Military Press 10 reps

Squat 10 reps

Pulls Ups to Failure

Inside Grip Chins to Failure

Dips to Failure

Core Crunches 4x75

    Reverse Crunches 4x75

    Abs twists 4x75

Wednesday

Endurance pack march 3 hours 30 minutes 61lb load

Thursday

1 Hour 35 minutes Continuous Swimming

Friday

Strength Workouts for load carrying and Core strength

1 Mile Run 8 Minute Pace

Dead lift 5 reps

Weighted Glute Ham Raise 5 reps

Weighted Lunges 10 reps

Turkish Get Ups 5 Minutes continuously

Perform the circuit 3-5 times, try and increase weight each week increase the load each time

Saturday

6 mile speed march 40 minutes with 21lb load record your best time

Sunday

1 hour 30 minutes speed marching in 31lb load

Stage 4 Week 20

3rd Progression Stage

Monday

Military Assault Circuit

Weighted Step Ups 3x12

Weighted Lunges 3x12

Box jumps between two boxes 3x12

Swiss Ball Pike 3x12

Burpee's 3x failure

Bench Press 4x6

Pull Ups x failure

Sprints 45 seconds sprinting with 1 minute rest repeat 8-10 times, rest 1 minute 30 seconds between circuits **add a weight vest to you workouts at 45lb weight**

Tuesday

Military Strength Endurance Training

Warm up with back extensions and running then perform the following with no more than 60 kg weight on the barbell, as many circuits as possible in 30 minutes then onto core work, session should last 45 minutes

Bench Press 10 reps

Military Press 10 reps

Squat 10 reps

Pulls Ups to Failure

Inside Grip Chins to Failure

Dips to Failure

Core Crunches 5x50

Reverse Crunches 5x50

Abs twists 5x50

Wednesday

Endurance pack march 3 hours 30 minutes 61lb load

Thursday

1 Hour 40 minutes Continuous Swimming

Friday

Strength Workouts for load carrying and Core strength

1 Mile Run 8 Minute Pace

Dead lift 5 reps

Weighted Glute Ham Raise 5 reps

Weighted Lunges 10 reps

Turkish Get Ups 5 Minutes continuously

Perform the circuit 3-5 times, try and increase weight each week increase the load each time

Saturday

6 mile speed march 60 minutes with 21lb load record your best time

Sunday

1 hour 30 Minutes speed marching in 31lb load

Stage 4 Week 21

3rd Progression Stage

Monday

Military Assault Circuit

Weighted Step Ups 3x12

Weighted Lunges 3x12

 Box jumps between two boxes 3x12

Swiss Ball Pike 3x12

Burpee's 3x failure

Bench Press 4x6

Pull Ups x failure

Sprints 45 seconds sprinting with 1 minute rest repeat 8-10 times, rest 1 minute 30 seconds between circuits **add a weight vest to you workouts at 45lb weight**

Tuesday

Military Strength Endurance Training

Warm up with back extensions and running then perform the following with no more than 60 kg weight on the barbell, as many circuits as possible in 30 minutes then onto core work, session should last 45 minutes

Bench Press 10 reps

Military Press 10 reps

Squat 10 reps

Pulls Ups to Failure

Inside Grip Chins to Failure

Dips to Failure

Core Crunches 5x60

     Reverse Crunches 5x60

     Abs twists 5x60

Wednesday

Endurance pack march 3 hours 30 minutes 61lb load

Thursday

1 Hour 45 minutes Continuous Swimming

Friday

Strength Workouts for load carrying and Core strength

1 Mile Run 8 Minute Pace

Dead lift 5 reps

Weighted Glute Ham Raise 5 reps

Weighted Lunges 10 reps

Turkish Get Ups 5 Minutes continuously

Perform the circuit 3-5 times, try and increase weight each week increase the load each time

Saturday

6 mile speed march 60 minutes with 21lb load record your best time

Sunday

1 hour 30 Minutes speed marching in 31lb load

Stage 5 Week 22

1st Test Stage record first attempt scores

Monday

8 Mile run best effort

Tuesday

Combat Swimming test

500m 12 minutes

25 m Underwater Swim repeats 4 times

Wednesday

 12 mile pack march to be completed in 4 hours 40 minutes

Thursday

Rest

Friday

Rest

Saturday

9 mile speed march 90 minutes with 21lb load record your best time

Sunday

Body weight test

100+ Press Ups 2 Minutes

100+ Sit Ups 2 Minutes

20+ Pull Ups

Stage 5 Week 23

1st Test Stage record second attempt scores

Monday

8 Mile run best effort

Tuesday

Combat Swimming test

500m 12 minutes

25 m Underwater Swim repeats 4 times

Wednesday

 12 mile pack march to be completed in 4 hours 40 minutes

Thursday

Rest

Friday

Rest

Saturday

9 mile speed march 90 minutes with 21lb load record your best time

Sunday

Body weight test

100+ Press Ups 2 Minutes

100+ Sit Ups 2 Minutes

20+ Pull Ups

Stage 6 Week 24

Final Endurance Test Week

Monday
8 Mile run best effort
Tuesday
Rest

Wednesday
30Mile Endurance March to be completed in 9 hours 40lb pack
Thursday
Rest
Friday
Rest
Saturday
9 mile speed march 90 minutes with 21lb load record your best time
Sunday
Rest

Thank you purchasing this book. You can read more and contact me via www.pnorthfitness.com.

www.ingramcontent.com/pod-product-compliance
Lightning Source LLC
Chambersburg PA
CBHW080756290526
45790CB00008B/3473